Ergonomics in the Dental Office

Ergonomics in the Dental Office

Susan S. Parker, RDH, MEd, MBA

Retired Associate Professor, Clinical Comprehensive Dentistry
Louisiana State University School of Dentistry
New Orleans, LA, USA

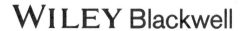

This edition first published 2022
© 2022 John Wiley & Sons, Inc.

Registered Office
John Wiley & Sons, Inc., 111 River Street, Hoboken, NJ 07030, USA

Editorial Office
111 River Street, Hoboken, NJ 07030, USA

For details of our global editorial offices, customer services, and more information about Wiley products visit us at www.wiley.com.

Wiley also publishes its books in a variety of electronic formats and by print-on-demand. Some content that appears in standard print versions of this book may not be available in other formats.

Library of Congress Cataloging-in-Publication Data applied for:
ISBN: 9781119131373 (paperback)

Cover Design: Wiley
Cover Images: Courtesy of Susan S. Parker

Set in 9.5/12.5pt STIXTwoText by Straive, Pondicherry, India

SKY10032451_011322

Contents

Preface

Occupational musculoskeletal disorders (MSDs) are a significant health and safety problem facing most workforces today. The basic **cause** of these MSDs is exposure to **risk factors to the worker**. When a worker is exposed to MSD risk factors, their body begins to tire and thus becomes fatigued. When the fatigue outruns the body's recovery system, a musculoskeletal imbalance happens to that body. Sometimes the worker has no indication that there is a problem developing. This sounds like it should be simple to change. However, the human body and the various styles of work that individuals do require some knowledge about the body and its various muscle groups to keep these musculoskeletal pains from developing.

One such occupation that is really physically tough on the human body is dentistry. Dental health providers are at an increased risk of work-related stress and musculoskeletal discomfort by the very nature of their daily work. In spite of different working patterns, there are parallel levels of symptoms in dentists and dental hygienists across nations. There are several links on the internet and journal articles addressing various ergonomic issues. However, there is a need for a more specific source of information for the entire dental health team that can be easily accessed and understood. Risk factors for MSDs are multifactorial. Therefore, the goal of this short book is to describe the causes of the musculoskeletal problems that might be occurring daily in the dental office and that we might have no idea are occurring, and to outline solutions to them. Symptoms appear very early in some dental careers, with a surprisingly higher prevalence of MSDs found in educational training.

The book aims to be easily accessible and to address specific ergonomic issues that might arise for dental practitioners in the operatory or working environment in the dental office. This information should be able to enlighten anyone who might need help in understanding how the body can be misused and the importance of ergonomics in most if not all walks of life. The desired outcome is a comprehensive strategy for mitigation and an integration of practices to reduce most ergonomic risks, in order to achieve amelioration in workplace ergonomics for employee health and safety. Efforts to address this problem for all dental professionals need to take an interdisciplinary, progressive approach. Prevention is better than treatment. Though no one can go back and make a brand new start, anyone can start from where they are and create a brand new ending. Let us begin now to appreciate our miraculous body and its human engineering.

As Mahatma Gandhi said, "The future depends on what you do today."

Acknowledgments

I would like to thank all of my wonderful dental students and many others who encouraged me in this endeavor. First, I would like to thank Wiley publishing and the many brilliant people there who worked with me on this publication Erica Judisch, Tanya McMullin, Susan Engelken, Bhavya Boopathi, Angela Cohen, and Dr. Sally Osborn. My gratitude to Mr. Rick Ames Blanchette for coming to New Orleans to meet me and to give me this opportunity.

My dear family, colleagues and friends who helped me in every way and listened – Brandi Windham, Muscular Therapist, Dr. Frank Martello, Dr. Doug Dederich, Dr. Stephanie Noe, Shelly Zagor, Paul Caballero, Shelly Downs, Sharon Hearn, Curt Hearn, and the late Don Farnworth. Thank you all from the bottom of my heart.

1

What Is Ergonomics?

Let's start with some definitions of key terms. The terms "human-factors engineering" and "ergonomics" are used interchangeably on the North American continent. In Europe, Japan, and most of the rest of the world, the prevalent term used is ergonomics. *Merriam-Webster* (n.d.) defines ergonomics as "(1) an applied science concerned with designing and arranging things people use so that the people and things interact most efficiently and safely - called the biotechnology, human engineering, human factors"; and "(2) the design characteristics of an object resulting especially from the application of the science of ergonomics." The *Britannica Online Encyclopedia* defines human-factors engineering as ergonomics or human engineering (Holstein & Chapanis, 2018). The term "human-factors engineering" is used equally to designate a body of knowledge, a process, and a profession. Human engineering is a science dealing with the application of information on physical and psychological characteristics to the design of devices and systems for human use.

The word "ergonomics" is derived from the ancient Greek *ergon*, which means work, and *nomos*, which means law. Ergonomics can also be seen as the science concerned with how to fit a job to a person's anatomical, physiological, and psychological characteristics in a way that will enhance human efficiency and thus contribute to a safer working environment. The discipline of ergonomics was formalized after the end of World War II. The science of ergonomics looks for ways to make work easier on a worker's body by using a combination of techniques and equipment that will prevent injuries while maintaining efficiency.

Human-factors engineers have tried to show that with appropriate techniques it is possible to identify human-made mismatches and thus to find workable solutions to these mismatches through the use of methods developed in the behavioral sciences. Design decisions and approaches cannot be reached without a lot of trial and error. The telephone and the typewriter keyboard are but two out of thousands of examples that might have been selected to show how human-factors engineering has been consciously applied to solve technological problems. Today,

Ergonomics in the Dental Office, First Edition. Susan S. Parker.
© 2022 John Wiley & Sons, Inc. Published 2022 by John Wiley & Sons, Inc.

we can just look at the many advances in the US space program, automotive industry, computer technology, and more. More broadly, in every sector globally there is a realization that physical problems occur because of workplace setups that can cause misalignment of the human anatomy, and thus physical pain and mental misery. The list continues to expand as the world moves at a faster and faster pace and there is a realization that ergonomics is essential in daily life.

In the January 2021 edition of *Costco Connection*, there is a short article on how to prevent and recover from bad work habits. We are reminded to commit to healthy work habits such as sitting tall and getting up every hour to move that body. We must begin to listen to our bodies. Researchers have used a number of methods to measure these musculoskeletal disorders (MSDs) or imbalances, yet these are really just subjective. Gravity is the one force that affects all existence and behavior on earth. Defining and maintaining a steady center of gravity is therefore important and the most significant natural step in accomplishing any given task. Each individual has their own unique center of gravity. We can collaborate with other people and disciplines in order to achieve a better understanding of what needs to happen to avoid an MSD, but ultimately it is our individual responsibility to learn to treat our body with kindness.

The practice of dentistry today

From the vantage point of the twenty-first century we can see a continuous pattern of musculoskeletal strain and awkward postures among dental providers and their auxiliaries. A combination of unsupported postures, excessive movements, and repetitive motions explains the evolution of MSDs in the practice of dentistry. Sitting down has not been the golden panacea that it was once thought to be. The human spine and its musculature constitute a living structure that benefits from movement. Our spinal disks must have motion in order to be nourished. Any attempt to constrain the spine will be met with failure and pain. Low back pain is one of the leading MSDs for dental practitioners. This is directly related to too much sitting.

After teaching ergonomics to dental students for many years, I began to see that something more was needed in the dental curriculum to address this problem. We need to look for better practitioner positioning as we practice. Within the last decade, 47 percent of US dental schools have indicated that ergonomics is a very important part of the dental curriculum. Some dental schools have made ergonomics an elective if the dental curriculum cannot be expanded further, so that the study of ergonomics is at least available to dental and dental hygiene students. Students of dentistry and dental hygiene should begin to envision **ergonomic awareness** as an angel (the subconscious mind) that lifts us (the practitioners) into a balanced posture when our conscious minds do not remember to do so

(Figure 1.1). This is an **imperative** part of the dental curriculum. It is never too early to raise students' awareness of ergonomic principles for dental practitioners and the consequences that can result from practicing without using this ergonomic knowledge. It is important as a preventive measure as well. It is a known fact that we stimulate the same brain regions when we visualize doing something as when we actually do it physically. It is so very important for dental students and hygienists to learn their individual **neutral position** when working on a patient. This is how ergonomics needs to be taught. Once an understanding of it is generally accepted and understood, the process of incorporating knowledge of ergonomics into the dental curriculum will be a lot easier and much more natural to each student. Thomas Edison said, "There is a better way for everything. Find it!" It is the quality, not the quantity of life that matters.

One must remember that the body is a machine consisting of optics, mechanics, chemistry, and electronics. The key factor in maintaining musculoskeletal health is maintaining the body's neutral position as much as possible during the day. What is this neutral position? The **neutral position** (or **comfort zone**) is defined as the position of an appendage that is neither moved away from nor directed toward the body's midline, nor laterally twisted (Figure 1.2). There is always a

Figure 1.1 Ergonomic awareness.

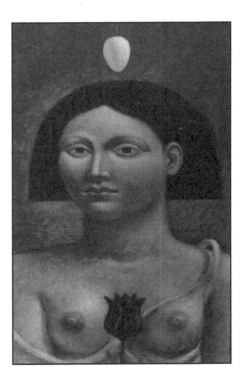

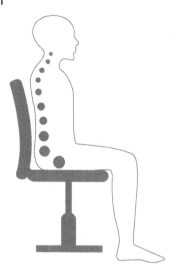

Figure 1.2   Neutral position.

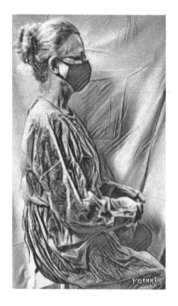

Figure 1.3   Neutral position for the registered dental hygienist.

neutral zone for every joint and muscle. An individual must keep their entire musculature evenly balanced. Our posture and how we habitually use our body the most are what can lead our body and spine to begin to shorten and to curve into unhealthy patterns. Keeping the spine healthy at every age is crucial to the general health and longevity of the physical body.

How a dental practitioner stands, walks, and uses their feet can lock patterns into the feet, ankles, knees, and hips. The key is movement – *this* is the goal of the practitioner. We must keep the body in motion as much as we can during our daily dental work. The neutral position is key and encompasses a deeper journey for the practitioner, in that the sides of the body are released (Figure 1.3), thus freeing the "stuck ribs" that ultimately shorten the body, resulting in the ribcage and head becoming "weighed down" on the lower body. The abdominal muscles must be strong, as they play such an important role in connection to the health of the back and spine. Strong gluteal muscles are important as well to help the individual attain this personal neutral position.

2

Musculoskeletal Disorders

In 2001, the Bush administration announced voluntary guidelines to reduce occupational repetitive-stress injuries in the "shortest possible time." The Occupational Health and Safety Administration (OSHA) Administrator at that time, John Henshaw, made a promise that his agency would immediately begin work on industry- and task-specific guidelines to reduce musculoskeletal disorders (MSDs). "We know one size does not fit all," he stated. The intention was to build on evidence-based best practices already developed and to use the best available science in dealing with ergonomic injuries. This four-phased approach included an enforcement arm targeting "bad actor" employers under a legislative authority known for requiring employers as a general duty to maintain safe and healthy work sites. "Our goal is to help workers by reducing ergonomic injuries in the shortest possible time," stated the then Labor Secretary, who considered the plan an improvement over the old rules because of its intention, which was to prevent ergonomic injuries before their occurrence. The program was designed and intended to reach a much larger number of "at-risk" workers.

The American Dental Association (ADA) offered testimony and written comments on ergonomic issues related to dentistry at a 2002 OSHA forum held at Stanford University. Yet this conclusion was based on subjective research. Currently, ergonomics is enforced under the "General Duty Clause" to report employers that subject workforces to ergonomics hazards. For further information on compliance with OSHA regulation, contact your state's local OSHA office.

In 2004, OSHA and the ADA recognized the value of establishing a collaborative relationship to foster safer and more healthful workplaces in the US. Their alliance's intention was to use their collective expertise in fostering a culture of prevention while sharing technical knowledge in ergonomics.

Later that year, the ADA presented an introduction to ergonomic risk factors, MSDs, approaches and interventions. The primary occupational risk factors for MSDs were reported as being repetition, mechanical stresses, posture, vibration,

Ergonomics in the Dental Office, First Edition. Susan S. Parker.
© 2022 John Wiley & Sons, Inc. Published 2022 by John Wiley & Sons, Inc.

cold temperature, and extrinsic strain. It is very important to be aware and to make clear that each of these risk factors alone is not the direct cause of a particular MSD, as any MSD is more likely be attributed to multiple risk factors. This multi-factorial problem is sometimes referred to as cumulative trauma disorder (CTD). Some literature defines this as an "acute elevation of micro trauma that happens to the body in an insidious way at a rate faster than the body can repair." Carpal tunnel syndrome is included as a CTD, for instance.

One systematic review of 23 studies revealed the prevalence of MSDs among dentists and dental hygienists: 70 percent of dental workers in the research experienced pain in the hand and wrist. It is easily apparent why MSDs are prevalent in the dental profession. Dentists and hygienists are required to perform physically demanding work in prolonged static postures, using the muscles of their arms and hands almost continuously throughout the day. As a result of working in the same position for prolonged periods of time, dental professionals and dental students are very likely to cause injury to their musculoskeletal systems.

Now just consider the procedures performed by the dental hygienist every day (Figure 2.1). In a typical working day, dental hygienists do probing, scaling, root planning, cleaning, polishing, and flossing teeth, with the use of their hands and wrists and usually without rest breaks in between. All of these are repetitive in nature. In addition, when these are done in a workstation that is not set up properly for the individual practitioner, the chance of developing repetitive injuries is multiplied. A common fallacy is that if a design is satisfactory for one person, then it is automatically satisfactory for everybody. Work done with arms above shoulder height and forceful movement of arms while working have been found to be statistically associated with work-related MSD symptoms in the lower shoulder and forearm.

RDH magazine reported that millions of dollars in income are lost every year when patient appointments must be canceled due to a dental practitioner being prevented from working because of pain as a result of an MSD. Economics and ergonomics are in alignment, in that safe and productive work will cost a company less in the long run. We are fortunate to be moving in the right direction here.

Lower back problems, herniated disks, upper back discomfort, neck pain, tendonitis, carpal tunnel syndrome, high muscle tension on the trapezoids, and pain in the lower extremities are just some of the MSDs reported by over 50 percent of dental workers. MSDs have many possible etiologies, some of which are poor posture, static posture, repetitive motion, mental stress, lack of physical fitness, genetic inclination, less flexibility, and lack of rest – and there are more. Even with the use of ergonomically, well-adjusted equipment on the rise, the literature reports an increase in back, neck, shoulder, and arm pain in up to 81% of dental professionals.

A research study by the National Institutes of Health found that a lack of significant emphasis on ergonomic principles can be one of the reasons for low levels of awareness and implementation of practices. Another evidence-based research

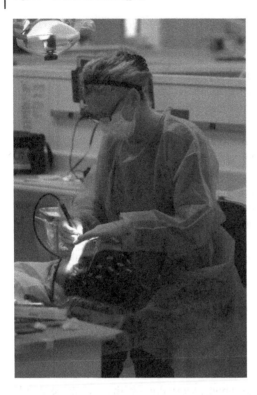

Figure 2.1 Dental hygienists perform many tasks that make them susceptible to repetitive injuries.

study conducted in India regarding ergonomics in clinical dentistry named some of the important and most prevalent MSDs in full- or part-time dental practitioners. Not surprisingly, these were low back pain, neck pain, pain in the wrist and hand joints, and shoulder pain.

Back pain is usually a composite of pain sent from points both above and below where the discomfort is felt. A key to successfully treating back pain is to track the components of the pain. The fact that there are so many different muscles associated with the spine can make this difficult. To simplify the process, picture the muscles as the outer and inner layers of the spine. The outer layers are the superficial spinal muscles or long muscles running parallel to the spine. The inner layers are the deep spinal muscles that are very short and originate diagonally to the spine. This angular arrangement gives them good working leverage for twisting and side-bending the spine. These muscles working together help to extend the spine.

One other published study measured perceived musculoskeletal symptoms among dental students in the clinical work environment. This study investigated the clinical tasks that place students at physical risk and the relationship between those tasks and musculoskeletal symptoms. A total of 61 percent (358/590) of students reported that they had experienced musculoskeletal symptoms related to their clinical work at the dental school. Of those students' symptoms, the neck represented 48 percent, the shoulder 31 percent, the back 44 percent, and the hands 20 percent (p<0.001). One national dental hygiene survey was done in 2012 via a poll that had 1210 respondents from 47 states and 6 provinces. One specific finding was that 65 percent worked more than 31 hours a week. Among the respondents, 36 percent reported at least one injury and 53.1 percent of the others used over-the-counter medication. The primary injury sites among the dental hygienists who responded to the survey were the neck, the shoulders, and the mid and upper back. As a direct result of an injury, 38 percent of practitioners had been forced to reduce their work hours permanently.

Multiple treatment options exist for the management of pain, but it is important to remember that all interventions should be intended to prevent or minimize musculoskeletal pain. A specialist or physician should be consulted and a thorough physical examination and assessment of the individual done prior to intervention or treatment. Dentistry is a wonderful profession. Therefore, we must keep striving to find out as much as we can to make it safer for actively practicing dental professionals.

Occupational Safety and Health Administration

Federal laws on ergonomics in the USA can be difficult to interpret due to the complexity of workplace safety regulations. OSHA began to look into ergonomics in 1970 because of the job-related injuries reported, but it was not until 1990 that OSHA established an Office of Ergonomics Support. In 2001, after Congress used an obscure law to block introduction of OSHA's ergonomic standards from 2000, OSHA turned to a broader rule to enforce safe practices: the General Duty Clause of 1970. Section 5(a)(1) of the General Duty Clause requires employers to keep facilities "free from recognized hazards" that are causing or are likely to cause death or serious physical harm to employees. Today, OSHA uses this General Duty Clause to sanction employers that subject workers to ergonomic hazards. However, the clause is a fairly blunt legal tool in that it requires a high burden of proof.

In 2001 OSHA announced voluntary guidelines to reduce occupational repetitive-stress injuries "in the shortest possible time." As stated previously, its goal is to reduce ergonomic injuries in the shortest possible time by helping to prevent these injuries before they occur, and to reach a much larger number of "at-risk" workers. OSHA recognizes that "one size does not fit all," but promises the best available science in dealing with the problem of ergonomic injuries. Determination of whether an MSD is "work related" requires different approaches tailored to specific workplace conditions and exposures. MSDs currently account for a full third of all injury and illness cases in the USA.

All dental employers are mandated to provide a safe workplace. OSHA coverage for a workplace facility encompasses two major requirements: training and record keeping. Employers with 11 or more employees (including part-time and temporary employees) must maintain records of employee reports of MSDs, MSD signs and symptoms, MSD hazards, and employer responses to such reports. In addition, OSHA's remit includes job hazard analyses, hazard control measures, quick-fix processes, ergonomic program evaluations, work restrictions, and time off work, together with healthcare professionals' opinions. Since OSHA's General Duty Clause extends well beyond known hazards and gives inspectors far-reaching authority to cite a facility for any workplace hazard, the **OSHA Dental Manual** provides extensive coverage of what to do to prepare for an OSHA site visit. The blood-borne pathogens standards, dental infection control guidelines, a medical waste storage/disposal protocol, and revised hazard communication standards under the new Globally Harmonized System (GHS) are explained and illustrated. A "do-it-yourself" kit simplifies the task of writing numerous safety plans. The history of OSHA has shown that operations will not be targeted as long as they address any ergonomic hazards. Between 2009 and 2011, OSHA only issued three ergonomics citations under the General Duty Clause. This limited attack on ergonomic hazards is due to the high burden of proof associated with this clause.

Because of the COVID-19 pandemic that began in early 2020, OSHA added a section on control and prevention. The current OSHA guidance for dentistry and dental employers is not regulatory, but contains recommendations as well as existing mandated safety and health standards for dental workers at increased risk for COVID-19 infection due to occupational exposure. OSHA has stated that dental employers should adopt infection prevention and control strategies based on the individual workplace hazard assessment, using combinations of engineering and administrative controls, safe work practices, and personal protective equipment (PPE) to prevent worker exposures. The Centers for Disease Control and Prevention have also developed interim COVID-19 guidance for all employers and businesses. OSHA and the US Department of Health and Human Services provide joint guidance for all employers on preparing workplaces for COVID-19. The American Dental Hygienists Association supported a recent study to estimate the prevalence of COVID-19 infection among US dental hygienists and to describe infection prevention and control procedures for them. The conclusions of this study as of October 2020 indicated that the estimated prevalence rate of COVID-19 in dental hygienists who participated in the study was low. However, a need for further support for dental hygienists was seen in the areas of PPE and mental health. These are critical issues that need to be studied and addressed continually.

Currently OSHA manuals for training and compliance for the dental office are available for purchase online or to download. They can be found on the US Department of Labor website specific to OSHA (www.bls.gov).

3

Positioning for Success

The dental work environment and its characteristics can be represented by four domains. In a study by Khan and Chew (2013), sitting position, instrument handling, use of dental loupes or no use, and frequency of working hours were examined, with 410 clinical-year dental students participating. Students who used a comfortable work stool with back support were far less likely to have lower back pain. Regarding handling of instruments, work that was done with arms raised above shoulder height and the forceful movement of arms were found to be statistically associated with musculoskeletal disorder (MSD) symptoms in the lower shoulder and the forearm. Interestingly, the study reached no statistically significant findings in relation to the use of loupes and prevalence of discomfort in the neck and upper back. This might be as a result of the level of the participating dental students, as D1 students usually begin clinical learning in simulation labs. Findings from another evidence-based research article from the *Journal of IMAB* in 2012 support the argument for integrating ergonomics for students into the dental curriculum.

I have addressed the problems associated with the practice of dentistry and dental hygiene, namely MSDs because of repetitive motion involving high-finesse dental procedures and the precision needed, along with control of the instruments used in these various dental procedures. Optimally, the success of dental work involves working conditions for the dentist and the dental team that are within a sound ergonomic environment. Ergonomics in dentistry hones in on the working posture of the dental practitioner, be it dentist, dental hygienist or assistant.

Posture

Posture is the main key for prevention of MSDs. Posture in ergonomics means the manner in which different parts of the body are located to execute a particular task. In dentistry, there is a spatial arrangement of the working position of the operator's body around the patient lying in the dental chair. The ideal posture for the dentist provides optimal working conditions (access, visibility, and control while working in the patient's mouth) and physical and psychological comfort throughout clinical dental work. A good working position reduces stress and muscular tension and provides comfort, lack of pain, and a lower risk of errors that do contribute to MSDs (head hanging too low, shoulders slumped forward, no core support by practitioner, tight body, elbows above forearms, etc.). The dental operator's spine must maintain its natural curves, specifically of the cervical, thoracic, and lumbar spine when seated, which in turn should help to preserve the lower back curve. Appropriate back support is critical to help reduce the occurrence of low back pain, as well as the practitioner having strong core muscles. Backrests and lumbar support are just one of multiple ergonomic considerations when selecting an operator stool. Other ergonomic features need to be carefully assessed to determine that the particular operator chair in use will contribute to the health and career longevity of the dental healthcare provider. Some of these additional features are armrests, seat material, casters, and cylinder height, just to name a few.

A **balanced posture** or neutral position should be the definitive reference point for the working postures used daily by the dentist or dental hygienist. When the dentist deviates from this balanced posture, be it from habit, work routine, or poorly designed workstations, problems can emerge (Figure 3.1). Unequal

(a)   (b)

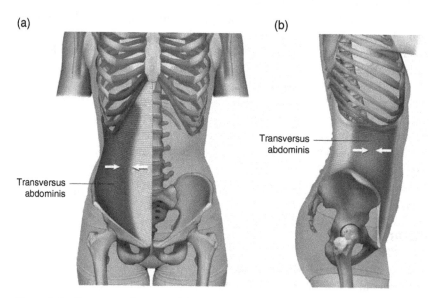

Figure 3.1 Transverse abdominis. The action of this muscle compresses the abdomen to support the abdominal viscera against the pull of gravity. Courtesy of Dr. Joe Muscolino.

distribution of the dental practitioner's body weight can lead to muscle imbalances, which lead to MSDs. The result may be vertebral muscular pain, which may limit the ability to practice. Dental practitioners must not ignore their own body and its adaptive limits. The correct balanced working posture is recommended to be maintained within the limits imposed by conditions of practice throughout all stages of clinical work. This neutral position is the result of ergonomic studies adapted to the needs of dental procedures.

Strong core muscles and maintaining a spinal curve are also essential to the **prevention** of pain. Strong transverse abdominal muscles are effective in reducing the chance of low back pain. The transverse abdomens is the deepest of the three anterolateral wall muscles (Figure 3.2). It is functionally important for core (powerhouse) stabilization. Think of it as the corset muscle. The neutral torso position is based on evenly balancing the practitioner's weight on the chair seat, with elbows close to the sides of the body and no more or less than 20 degrees away from the body, at the level of the patient's mouth. This balanced posture involves a tall back and a respect for body symmetry, with a forward inclination of the trunk of a maximum of 20 degrees and a forward inclination of the head of up to 20–25 degrees from the trunk (Figure 3.3). The dental practitioner must maintain the body's neutral position to preserve musculoskeletal health. The spine is supported by bony vertebrae and little stress, if any, is placed on the muscle and ligaments when in a neutral position. This posture should be comfortable and thus maintain a natural postural balance. A helpful analogy when teaching students is also to have the individual student envision a beautiful silk cord attached to the top of the head, holding up the head and reaching to the heavens with the chin parallel to the ground. Dental practitioners should learn mindful approaches to help maintain

Figure 3.2 Deviation from correct working position.

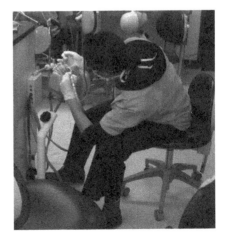

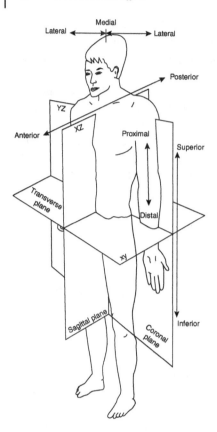

Figure 3.3 Planes of the body.

this correct positioning throughout the day so that they do not fall back into old patterns. Here it is **always** very important to remember that the ears should be over or above the shoulders as well. Many years ago Tai chi masters introduced an image of a silk cord attached to the top of the head to keep the head in the correct position, and this visual is still used today because it works. Also today there are companies that sell postural shirts or electronic patches that alert the practitioner to excessive forward bending or any deviation from neutral position.

Postural symmetry means all body horizontal lines being parallel and perpendicular to the median line of the body (Figure 3.4). The dental work environment is represented by four domains: sitting position, instrument handling, use or nonuse of dental loupes, and frequency of working hours. Preserving a balanced posture throughout clinical work is largely dependent on the dentist and the intraoral working field. Ideally, the surface of the treated teeth should be parallel to the front of the dentist. The dental clinician should always try to face the patient directly during dental treatment. The recommendation is that the distance between the

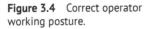

Figure 3.4 Correct operator working posture.

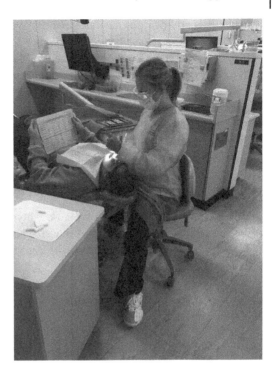

working field and the dentist's eyes is 35–40 cm, or slightly more for taller dentists. To maintain this ideal posture throughout the day, the working equipment and the working space or workstation must be tailored to the individual dentist and fit "like a glove." Instruments should be kept within a 53 cm radius of the dental assistant to minimize the need to reach or twist. The dental workstation comprises the dental stool, the patient lying in the anatomical chair, the dental unit and its components, and the fixed elements surrounding the workstation. The overhead light should be positioned slightly behind and to one side of the dental clinician's head. This will minimize shadowing effects. The optimal lightweight head-mounted light can alternatively be the best ergonomic choice.

Seating

An operator's choice of seating is critical and can help to make it a little easier for the dental practitioner to maintain a balanced posture. Therefore, dental practitioners should make the best choice for themselves. I always suggest trying out different chairs to see what fits the individual. Just because a chair may be ergonomically designed, does not mean that it cannot hurt the practitioner if it is not adjusted properly or right for that person. A variety of chairs offering different methods for sitting are available today (Figure 3.5). There are "ergonomic" chairs, which still need to be properly adjusted for use by the individual practitioner. A true waterfall design, while just one of the many concepts in ergonomic seating, is an essential principle (Figure 3.6). The waterfall front or design for dental hygienists helps to prevent users' legs from being pinched or losing circulation. The dental professional's chair must be designed so that the seating position can be slightly elevated beyond parallel without restricting blood flow to the legs. This allows the operator to maintain a forward and upward posture while operating and transfers some of the body's support to the feet, referred to as "leg-balanced" seating. There are eight keys to selecting the proper stool (www.desergo.com):

- Cast star base construction with high-quality casters and bearings. This allows the operator to move and to improve visual access.
- A fully adjustable hydraulic gas lift to accommodate the wide assortment of patient sizes and restrictions.
- A true waterfall design.
- Quick, simple, and easy-to-use adjustments.
- A strong forward base-tilt capacity.

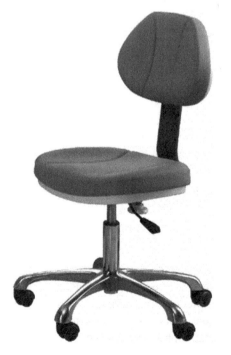

Figure 3.5　Standard dental chair.

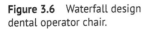

Figure 3.6 Waterfall design dental operator chair.

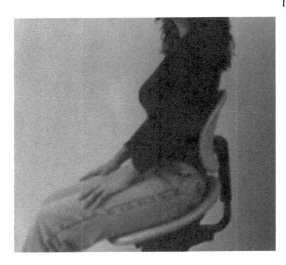

- Strong lumbar support without shoulder impingement.
- Firm and supportive seating surfaces.
- Options for personalization, including the capability to add highly supportive arms that function through a wide range of motion.

It is critical here to state once again that the individual practitioner must understand that their height plays a very important role in their choice of dental seating. Some manufacturers use a standard height to develop their products, and of course this has negative consequences for practitioners who are not the "standard" height. For example, I am 5'9" tall and I had to learn the hard way that the teaching I had been given on seating in the operatory in dental hygiene school worked against my body type. Consequently, it did not take long before knee issues began to surface for me at the beginning of my clinical practice. For instance, the thighs should *not* be parallel to the floor for most people, they should slope down so no pressure is placed on the knees. This also helps to maintain the lower back curvature.

Saddle stools offer many benefits for the practitioner (Figure 3.7). The saddle opens the hip angle and positions the operator closer to the patient. The use of a stool is somewhat akin to supported standing. Another company promotes "zen wave" technology, which provides for pelvis rotation forward and optimal pressure point dispersion. The feel is akin to "floating on water." Also there are sit-and-stand dental stools, which aid and support proper spinal alignment, as dentistry requires a forward/declined posture. Longer-legged operators need especially to assess the height of the chair or stool so that the hip angle is correct and the pelvis is in a position that facilitates the lower spinal curve. Sometimes a

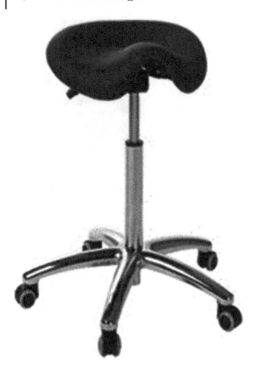

Figure 3.7 Saddle stool.

lumbar pillow support can help keep this problem at bay, but never underestimate the power of a strong core. The knees should not touch the seat of the patient chair and the weight must be evenly distributed through the thighs, with both feet resting firmly on the floor. Ideally, there should be about 20 cm between the patient's chair and the practitioner's stool or chair. Armrests also can be very helpful in reducing strain for all practitioners.

I would be remiss if I did not mention stability balls (Figure 3.8). The principle is that since a stability exercise ball is "unstable," it then "forces" the practitioner to maintain balance through "active sitting." The idea is that this active sitting automatically encourages proper spinal alignment and thus helps to signal the core muscles (transverse abdominis) to engage. Another benefit is that the dynamic movement and sway do enhance the practitioner's circulation and boost their energy. The ball is height adjustable. The absence of a backrest may further promote active sitting and strengthen the abdominal muscles if used correctly. One disadvantage I see with the stability ball is the lack of lumbar support, unless the operator has a strong core and can maintain balance and the natural lower back curve while performing dental procedures.

When positioning the patient, it is important to keep in mind the design of the dental patient chair. Make sure to select a chair with a thin back. This will allow the clinician close access to the patient, so that the clinician's legs can straddle the chair or go under

Figure 3.8 Stability ball.

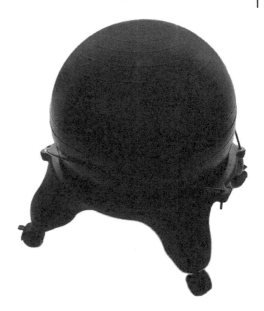

it without compromising the neutral position/balanced posture. Of course, it is important for the patient chair to be comfortable too. An adjustable headrest can make a world of difference for visibility of the dental worker as well as for comfort to the patient. The level of the dental worker's elbows should be even or level with the patient's mouth, with the elbows reaching 20 degrees or less away from the midline of the practitioner's body. Patients are usually very happy to accommodate the practitioner with movements of their head for the particular area the clinician is working on. The ideal working positions for the dental provider are the 9, 11, and 12 o'clock positions (Figure 3.9), because when in these positions a balanced posture is easier to keep without moving the upper body. Dental operators who deliver most of their treatment from the 10 o'clock position seem to experience more musculoskeletal problems.

To avoid straining the upper body and thus provide easier access to the individual tooth anatomy, the depth of the seat should support your thighs and allow three fingers' width behind the back of the knee with your back against the back rest.

Visibility

Today with the availability of magnification through loupes, the clinical microscope, the endoscope, and coaxial illumination (headlights), dental practitioners are better able to visualize the treatment area. Magnification assists with greater visibility to improve the field of vision and to help facilitate ideal postural positioning for musculoskeletal health.

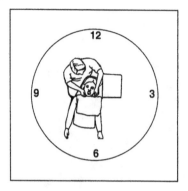

Figure 3.9 Ideal clock positions for dental work.

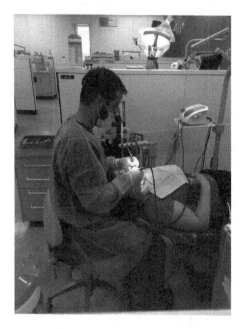

Figure 3.10 Loupes.

Loupes are well-known throughout the dental community today and evidence-based studies have proven ergonomic benefits as well as protection for the eyesight (Figure 3.10). Also now, with touch-free headlights, the risk of cross-contamination has been reduced. Bear in mind that the loupes must be properly measured to be of benefit to the dental practitioner. Too many times I have witnessed a dental student wearing loupes that were not properly measured, where the forward angle of the head was greater than the suggested 20–25 degrees from the trunk.

4

Instrumentation Techniques

Dental instruments are a direct extension of the practitioner's skill. Instrument manufacturing is an exacting skill. Fortunately, today we have exceptional companies that manufacture dental instruments of the highest standard and quality. We have seen in the industry a spirit of innovation that is exemplified by progressive concepts and improvements with new ideas. For example, carpal tunnel syndrome is a significant risk for dental hygienists, and thankfully the instrument companies continue to research ways to make instrumentation more ergonomically friendly. Dental instruments are organized according to their use or are "area specific." Each discipline – general dentists, endodontists, periodontists, oral surgeons, and pediatric dentists – has its own procedure-specific instruments.

Performance Logic in Clinical Dentistry, published by the Center for Human Performance in Dentistry, summarizes a human-centered path to health and success in dentistry. The five steps to peak performance are natural posture, patient positioning, stabilization and proper instrument delivery modalities, illumination, and operator balance and control of performance.

Practitioners' hands are integral to their work. As a direct result of sustained grips and prolonged awkward postures, dental professionals experience nearly four times the prevalence of hand, wrist, and arm pain than the general public. As dental tools have varied so much over time, we now know that the handle grip area on all tools should be at least 10 mm, although the ideal dental instrument weight has yet to be determined.

The dental practitioner should assess the site and visualize the anatomy of the tooth or teeth when selecting the instruments to be used for each dental procedure. The simplest grouping is to place the hand instruments for a certain procedure in sealed paper bags for sterilization. Cassettes have become invaluable as well for the private dental practitioner as well as for the dental school environment.

Ergonomics in the Dental Office, First Edition. Susan S. Parker.
© 2022 John Wiley & Sons, Inc. Published 2022 by John Wiley & Sons, Inc.

At this point I will emphasize the dental hygienist's armamentarium. Registered dental hygienists (RDHs) have specific set-ups for their dental tasks. A typical dental hygienist's armamentarium is composed of exam kits, nonsurgical maintenance kits, and periodontal kits, including Gracey curettes. Selection of instruments and how specific instruments are used have profound impacts on the RDH's musculoskeletal health – and therefore on the longevity of their practice. Ultrasonics and piezos have greatly reduced muscle tension and the resulting fatigue from hand scaling, although it should be stressed that hand scaling still needs to be done alongside the use of ultrasonics.

Finger rests

One very important technique taught in dental and dental hygiene programs is to use finger rests to stabilize the instrument while performing dental scaling or other types of dental work. To prevent the increased stress on the wrist and forearm tendons due to pinch force, a correct modified pen grasp must be maintained (Figure 4.1). The current environment during the COVID-19 pandemic does not advocate the use of aerosol-producing units, thus it is all the more important for the dental practitioner to properly utilize hand instrumentation only.

Finger rests may also reduce muscle stress and prevent injury due to muscle fatigue. One finger rest reduces thumb pinch force and muscle activity in most cases. Using finger rests plays an important role in reducing the muscle load on the hand and should be taught in the instrumentation labs at the beginning of the curricula.

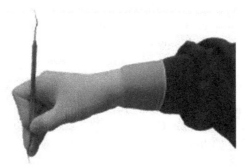

Figure 4.1 Pen grasp. The pen grasp of the instrument reduces stress on the wrists and forearms.

Selection of instruments

One goal in selecting instruments should be the compressibility in the grip area. Again, this will aid the hygienist in reducing pressure on the fingers and wrists and thus provide increased comfort when using the instrument.

The mouth is usually divided into four quadrants. There are anterior and posterior teeth, with mesial, distal, facial or buccal, lingual, and occlusal surfaces of each tooth. The tooth anatomy itself is complex, with roots, cementoenamel junction and developmental grooves. Each tooth has its own morphology. Fortunately, we have a selection of instruments that are purposefully designed for the specific area of the mouth to be instrumented. Dental hygienists explore around the tooth with light overlapping strokes and we attempt to reach the epithelial attachment. Instrumentation requires good hand skills and practice to be able to remove the deposits on the teeth with correct fulcrum pressure and working strokes. This is not easy, and posterior teeth can be quite a challenge. However, the RDH chooses the curette that is designed for the posterior teeth and uses the correct technique, with perhaps a two-finger fulcrum.

A root planing procedure with a Gracey curette adapts to the root of the tooth to access the pocket, where proper blade placement and stroke activation with firm pressure achieve the desired outcome. The Old Dominion University (ODU) or pigtail explorer is then used with very light pressure to be sure the area is smooth and free of calculus deposits and biofilms.

Instruments with straight shanks allow the RDH to use the adjacent tooth as a fulcrum, whereas instruments with curved shanks are not as easy to use. A fulcrum might be established several teeth away. Fulcrum pressure that equals lateral pressure creates safe, powerful working strokes. A relaxed grip together with proper instrumentation techniques will go a long way to help prevent injury.

Appropriate patient positioning must be achieved for maximum efficiency and deposit removal, as well as correct instrument sharpening as needed. Ceramic stones are my go-to choice, utilizing magnification for more success. A sharpening stone should be included in each scaling kit so as to sharpen the instrument as needed without excess removal of the metal surface of the blade.

Ultrasonics

Periodontal debridement encompasses all procedures where the intention is to restore the gingival tissues to optimal health. With the safe use and correct technique of ultrasonics (Figure 4.2), either magnetostrictive or piezoelectric, the dental

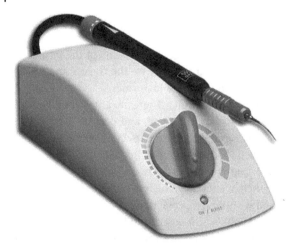

Figure 4.2 Ultrasonic.

practitioner's task is made a whole lot easier. Power scaling is a task that comprises a large part of a hygienist's day. However, if not done properly, damage can be caused to the tooth and root. "Less is more," as I always caution my students. Only low to medium power should be used with a light touch (pressure) and no "heavy hand." The instrument should be held near the working end with a modified pen grasp.

Today we have a variety of inserts. My usual go-to are Swivels and thin inserts with an extended shank or universal, as it is sometimes called. One company offers an insert specifically designed to help minimize neck, hand, and wrist fatigue. The Insight ultrasonic insert not only has a 360-degree swivel, but a dual-LED light added to it to enhance visibility.

Four-handed dentistry

In the 1960s a second person was added to the dental practice environment and the concept of "four-handed" dentistry became a reality. Having a dental assistant to handle instruments and manipulate patients' mouths can be *much* more efficient and effective for the practicing dentist. Dentistry has had to become more productive due to the advent of regulatory agencies, managed care, and quality assurance programs placing even greater demands on dental practitioners to provide a safe and comfortable environment for the patient and the working dental team.

Reclining dental chairs allow dentists and dental assistants to sit down to practice. Today this is the standard procedure.

Ideally, true four-handed dentistry is the methodology of a team of highly skilled clinical practitioners working together in an ergonomically designed environment to improve the productivity of the dental team, which will improve the quality of care given to the patient. This is working smarter and not harder.

There are a handful of dentists who became pioneers in research that really laid the groundwork for four-handed dentistry. The concept is based on a set of criteria that define the conditions under which efficiency can be attained, with the use of economy of motion and ergonomically designed equipment, which is positioned in advance of patient procedures. The objective is to minimize the number and magnitude of motions and thus conserve energy while the dental practitioner is working on the patient. A protocol is drawn up for every treatment and procedure. The dental practitioner should use the research that documents the principles of four-handed dentistry and follow through with equipment that meets these criteria.

Assisted dental hygiene has become a natural outcome of four-handed dentistry. Assisted dental hygiene is defined as one dental hygienist working out of two treatment rooms with a designated dental assistant. Again, by adding a valued team member, productivity and increased quality of care result. Another form of assisted dental hygiene practice is to utilize two dental hygienists and one dental assistant. This form or working requires a close-knit dental trio.

5

Office Equipment and Layout Design

As stressed throughout this book, maintaining proper posture is of the utmost importance in preventing musculoskeletal disorders among dental practitioners – dentists, dental hygienists, and dental assistants alike. Many practitioners have sustained injuries due to improper ergonomics that may be a direct effect of their work environment.

Operatory set-up and proper equipment are vital to maintaining health and achieving balanced posture – a neutral position. An ergonomically sound workstation should be a part of every dentist's and dental hygienist's armamentarium. Some elements that are included in the operatory set-up are the practitioners' chairs, the patient's chair, and the delivery system. Choosing the correct patient chair, the appropriate clinician chair, and the best delivery system is imperative to aid in maintaining proper posture and minimizing strain on the dental practitioner's back, neck, shoulders, and wrists.

There are several factors that can contribute to improper posture in operatory set-up, Including, but not limited to:

- Chairs being too low or too high.
- Inadequate lighting.
- Bracket table in the wrong location.
- Delivery system in the wrong location.
- Patient chair too wide, preventing dentist from getting into close proximity to the patient.
- Dentist's chair having little or no lumbar support.
- Dental assistant's chair having little or no arm and/or thoracic support.
- Practitioner's seat not padded or tilted slightly downward in the front to allow the hips to be higher than the knees.
- Backrest not fully adjustable with good lumbar support, or seat too tall and without lumbar support that is adjustable into the dental practitioner's lower back curvature.

Ergonomics in the Dental Office, First Edition. Susan S. Parker.
© 2022 John Wiley & Sons, Inc. Published 2022 by John Wiley & Sons, Inc.

The bottom line is to check for proper positioning of the dental patient before beginning the dental procedure. Recline the patient and adjust the patient headrest so that the occlusal plane is correct, and adjust the operator chair accordingly.

Delivery systems

The type of delivery system a dental clinician uses has a great impact on posture. There are a variety of delivery systems and each has its own pros and cons (Figure 5.1).

- The rear delivery system is the least expensive, and since it is behind the dentist, it keeps the equipment such as hand pieces and syringes out of the patient's view. While those features may be appealing to some, this system has restrictions that make it not the best ergonomic choice. If the dentist is practicing solo, extreme twisting, turning, extensive reaching, and leaning are required. This may also encourage eye strain, because the dentist has to turn away from the operating field to reach for the necessary hand pieces and instruments. In a rear delivery system the units are mounted in a fixed position, which also impedes the dental practitioners' free movement around the patient.
- The side delivery system is quite popular and is used in many dental offices and dental schools. Since the bracket tray, hand pieces, and air/water syringe are located on the side of the dentist's dominant hand, there is much less reaching, leaning, and trunk twisting required. This delivery system is the best when practicing solo (two-handed) dentistry. However, it may be difficult for the assistant to practice four-handed dentistry with this system.

Figure 5.1 Delivery systems for dental operators.

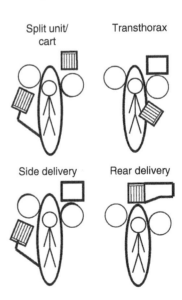

Split unit/ cart

Transthorax

Side delivery

Rear delivery

- The over-the-patient delivery system consists of a unit attached to an arm that is positioned over the patient's chest. This particular system can contribute to patient anxiety since the instruments are right in the patient's sight line. Additionally, the unit is susceptible to being bumped by patient movement.
- The over-the-head delivery system is a combination of rear delivery and over-the-patient delivery. With this system the dental practitioner is able to move freely around from the 7 o'clock to the 1 o'clock position.
- The transthorax delivery system is similar to the over-the-patient system. Instead of being placed directly over the patient's chest, the delivery system is positioned along the patient's left side. This type of delivery system is ideal for use in four-handed dentistry, because it enables the dental assistant to easily reach the hand pieces and instruments and thus transfer the needed instrument to the dentist while the dentist remains focused on the field of operation.

Chairs

The design and functionality of the patient's chair are as important as the right delivery system. It is important to have an ergonomically designed patient chair that allows the clinician to work comfortably.

Nevertheless, the most important chairs in the operatory are the dentist's and dental hygienist's chairs. Since the clinician is working 6–8 hours a day, the proper ergonomic features are critical for maximum health and thus minimum pain. There are countless types of chairs available and there are many features to consider when purchasing an operator chair, as discussed in Chapter 3.

Consultancy

As our knowledge of the importance of ergonomics in the dental office increases, several companies offer consultations and are available for hire to assist the dental practitioner in complete office design, from operatory to wet labs, from storage cabinets to patient waiting areas. These companies can be a great asset to help the practitioner determine the right equipment, chairs, and delivery systems that fit their needs. Ergonomic services are organizations that seek to create or sustain worker safety and health performance. US Ergonomics (www.us-ergo.com), ErgoFit Consulting (who also have a useful blog; www.ergofitconsulting.com), and individual consultants such as Dr. Lance Rucker (https://ergonomicsdental.com) provide services such as office equipment and layout evaluations, ergonomic practice assessment, integrated intervention planning, and follow-up.

6

Treating Patients with Disabilities

According to the US Centers for Disease Control and Prevention (CDC), approximately 53 million people in the USA – one in five – have a disability of some sort. About two-thirds of those disabilities are great enough to make everyday activities difficult and require the assistance of others. Dr. Frank Martello, a volunteer dentist for United Cerebral Palsy of Greater New Orleans for more than 30 years (Figure 6.1), has found that treating children and adults with intellectual and physical disabilities can be challenging and rewarding for everyone involved. He states that the key factor to remember is that *any* treatment one can provide will help to improve a patient's life. If the full range of treatment is not possible, even basic cleaning of the oral cavity will make your patient feel better. A cleaning can also decrease the potential foci of infection that can travel to all other parts of the body via respiratory, circulatory, and alimentary tracts.

Treating patients with disabilities presents a varied range of issues when it comes to seating (for both doctor and patient) and transferring from transportation to the office to the dental chair. Dr. Martello emphasizes the following when working on a patient with disabilities.

Know your patient

As with any patient, a current medical history is essential. This may have to involve the patient, their family, personal care attendants, physicians, and other medical professionals. Take note of any and all medications the patient may be using, especially if treatment requires that the patient be sedated. Listen to the people who attend to the patient on a daily basis.

Ergonomics in the Dental Office, First Edition. Susan S. Parker.

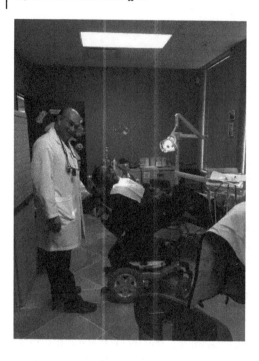

Figure 6.1 Dr. Frank Martello and patient.

Communication

Speak *to* your patient – never treat a patient, even if they are nonverbal, as a nonentity. Family and other caregivers who deal with the patient on a daily basis can serve as translators and help you streamline the treatment process. Typical patients with a mouthful of cotton roll, saliva ejectors, and dental instruments can communicate through expression and body language, and many severely disabled patients can as well.

A young woman who was injured in a crash was left with almost no muscle control and unable to speak. Her parents had not been taught how to clean her mouth. The patient listened to the dentist and she seemed agitated. Upon examination, food debris was found on her palate and in the vestibular areas of her mouth. Her parents were appalled to identify it as part of a meal from several days before. They were trying to brush her teeth, but didn't realize they weren't cleaning her whole mouth. They realized that her agitation was her way of alerting them to the issue. (There are unique toothbrushes to accommodate these problems. One is a toothbrush modified to "surround" the teeth to clean front, back, and biting surfaces (Figure 6.2).

Figure 6.2 Surround toothbrush.

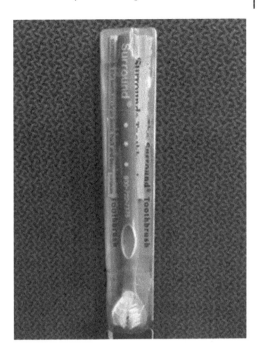

Put yourself in the patient's place – imagine what it would be like to be unable to take care of yourself and unable to tell others what the problem is. Then base your exam on what you would want done.

Access

The CDC also estimates that 6.5 million people use canes, walkers, or crutches and more than 2 million require a wheelchair for mobility and everyday tasks. The ideal dental practice is in a modern American with Disabilities Act (ADA)-compliant structure, with ramps, doorways, halls, and operatories that can accommodate wheelchairs and walkers. In the real world, adaptations can be made. Wheelchairs can be hauled up front door steps with enough people to do it safely, but a simple alternative is a pair of metal car ramps, available from any auto supply store. Wheelchair-bound patients should be pushed up the ramp and backed down the ramp. The person aiding the patient should always be between the wheelchair and any incline it might roll down.

Halls and operatories should be checked for anything that can impede passage, such as extension cords, mats, and dental equipment lines. It also helps to have the patient's hands and arms inside the chair, to avoid them getting caught on door frames, furniture, and such like. The operatory should have enough space around the chair to allow one or two people to assist the patient into the chair, and for emergency help should the need arise. Seating for a caregiver or family member is also needed and is more than just a courtesy. Their presence can calm an anxious patient, and they are undoubtedly an essential part of the treatment team.

Positioning

Depending on the patient's needs, seating adjustments will be required for both patient and doctor. For patients who are ambulatory, or using a walker or crutches, it may be a simple matter of raising or lowering the dental chair to the appropriate height. For nonambulatory patients, don't try to reinvent the wheel – simply ask the patient, family member, or other caregiver for the transfer method they routinely use to get the patient into other seating or a bed.

When transferring a patient from wheelchair to dental chair, the rule of thumb is **high to low**. This is especially true for patients with minimal muscle control. Let gravity help you conserve your energy and your back muscles by placing the dental chair lower than the wheelchair. Conversely, raise the dental chair higher to transfer the patient back to the wheelchair.

Patients with greater upper-body strength may find it easier to slide from wheelchair to dental chair, with both placed at the same level. Some wheelchairs can even raise and tilt, and can be used in place of the typical dental chair. This may require that the dentist and assistant adjust their chairs or even stand to provide treatment. Standing to provide treatment can be stressful. You can maximize your own comfort in this situation by using antifatigue mats.

Not all patients can be reclined once seated. Breathing and esophageal issues, shunts, spinal conditions, excess salivation, or reflux may prevent typical positioning. Have highly functioning suction ready at all times, even if the patient is seated completely upright.

Patients with postural problems may need help to be seated comfortably. There are catalogs and websites that offer a variety of assistive devices. If you do not have the time or budget to order from these resources, there are many simple items available at large retailers, such as:

- Small roll cushions, travel pillows, or "dog-bone" pillows for neck support.
- Wedge-shaped foam cushions, typically used for bed-bound patients.
- Small, lightweight synthetic fleece blankets – these can be rolled up into various configurations and held in shape with rubber bands or masking tape.

The most important feature of any posture aid is that it can be washed and is compatible with antibacterial sprays.

Restraints can be invaluable in treating patients with involuntary muscle movements. I have had patients who actually find comfort in having their uncontrollable movements minimized. This may be due to the effect of "lateral body pressure," as noted in research by Dr. Temple Grandin, a well-known autism spokesperson (https://www.autism.org/temple-grandin-inside-asd). However, informed consent prior to treatment with restraint is imperative, and rules addressing such restraint vary from state to state. Check with your state dental board for current rules and statutes pertaining to physical restraint.

Treatment for special needs patients

Patients with spasticity or poor muscle control will need help to "open wide." In addition to standard silicone bite blocks, there are numerous devices to prop the mouth open. One can engage the patient by asking them for their advice on brushing a plush animal's teeth. This can break the ice and a visual exam may then be done. Other patients may only allow an exam if they are standing up. Another may be willing to be seated, but won't open their mouth until their personal care attendant pats their cheek, puts both hands in their mouth to open it, and says, "Okay, let's do this!" As Dr. Martello states, sometimes four-handed dentistry takes six hands.

For patients who are on some form of sedation already, an increased dose may be sufficient to calm them enough to allow treatment to proceed. Usually family members and caregivers are very adept at judging dosages needed and the expected results from these doses. In more extreme cases, sedation and/or hospitalization may be required in order to do restorations or extractions. Not everyone is comfortable handling sedation cases in their practice – if this is the case, refer the patient to someone who is accustomed to such care.

The practice of dentistry generally takes a toll on the body, and accommodating patients with special needs can increase this impact. Long-term physical stress will limit the dental practitioner's well-being and productivity, so be aware and do take preemptive measures. Seat the patient in a position that is as comfortable for the practitioner as can be and at the same time suits the patient and their disability.

7

Exercise Disciplines and Alternative Therapies

There are many options to try that will help to alleviate the stress of dental work and a tired body, and to help each and every one of us to maintain the health and integrity of our physical body. It is such an exciting time in today's world. A growing amount of research confirms that in order to stay optimally healthy, the body needs to spend the bulk of its time doing what it was designed to do: move. We need to sit less and exercise more. The trick is finding the types of exercise that each person enjoys and eliminating those that do not contribute to a healthy body. Different forms of exercise give different types of energy and by listening to our body we can find what exercise works best for us.

The various modalities discussed in this chapter have stood the test of time and some do truly work to help us avoid musculoskeletal disorders. However, only the individual practitioner can cultivate this pull toward personal growth and body awareness through an absolute commitment to self and by living in the truth. Then and only then will the rewards of being healthy be ours. As the great poet Rilke stated, "The easy path leads to the hard life, but the hard path leads to the easy life."

Yoga

Yoga comes from the Sanskrit word *yunakti* meaning to yoke or to unite. It has been around for over 5000 years and is a group of physical, mental, and spiritual practices or disciplines that originated in ancient India. It leads to the union of individual consciousness, which indicates a perfect harmony between mind and body (www.mea.gov.in). Yoga does more than burn calories and tone muscles – it is a total mind–body workout that combines strengthening and stretching poses with deep breathing and meditation or relaxation. Yoga practice emphasizes the relationship of the breath and the spine. It is an integration of mind, breath, and

Ergonomics in the Dental Office, First Edition. Susan S. Parker.
© 2022 John Wiley & Sons, Inc. Published 2022 by John Wiley & Sons, Inc.

body, and enables you to listen to what your body is telling you. Yogic breathing is a unique method for balancing the autonomic nervous system.

There are over 100 forms of yoga. Some are fast paced and intense and others are gentle and relaxing. Yoga targets the arms, legs, glutes, and back, so it is a full-body workout. This increases flexibility and range of motion. It can also help to boost mood, as it relieves stress.

There is good reason for the dental practitioner to invest time in exploring yoga with a knowledgeable teacher who can teach the yoga poses. Tadasana ("mountain pose") is considered to be the starting point for practicing yoga postures or asanas. This is because this pose is closest to the anatomical position – the reference point for the study of movement and anatomy. Yoga improves posture because there is no stress to the muscles and the curve of the spine is preserved. I have been practicing yoga since the 1970s and I have never found a better form of exercise to ground me, to build muscle strength and balance, and to stretch. An added benefit is that I leave with a sense of peace and empowerment.

Here is a sampling of some yoga poses to help targeted body parts and alleviate pain. "Cat/cow" alternately opens the chest on the inhale and moved to a rounded and open back on the exhale. The spine, back, neck, shoulders, and hips are some of the areas that will be helped with this pose. Another easy pose is "eagle arms," which targets the wrists, arms, and shoulders. The practitioner wraps one arm under the other and crosses the forearms while pressing the palms together. When doing this pose, the arms should be at shoulder height and at a 90-degree angle. Side stretches are easy to do and stretch the arms, abs, waist, side of the body, and back. Another easy pose that helps to strengthen the arms, spine, back, lower abs, hamstrings, and lower back is the "sun salutation" with a fold and twist. While inhaling, reach the arms up overhead and connect the palms, then on the exhalation drop arms down and around with a twist to the left, bringing the right arm onto the left knee. Inhale, come back to center, and repeat the movement on the other side. There are many poses and as many adjustments that can be done. YouTube has many instructional videos for yoga. Remember only to do what feels right and that each individual is different, so what is good for some may not be for others. As a clinician you will be able to find a quiet spot during their workday or at lunch and just do child's pose. Relax into this posture and breath slowly in and out. You will find a certain peace of mind and body in the middle of the hectic workday.

Tai chi

Tai Chi as it is practiced in the West today can best be thought of as a moving form of yoga and meditation combined (Figure 7.1). There are a number of forms, which consist of a sequence of movements. Many of these movements are

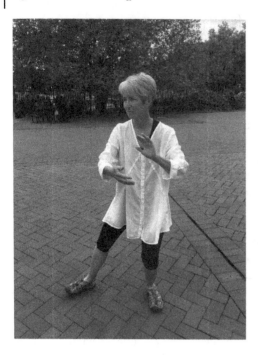

Figure 7.1 The practice of tai chi contributes to health and balance in our daily life.

originally derived from the martial arts. In tai chi movements are performed slowly, softly, and gracefully while breathing naturally, with even transitions between the movements. It is a truly meditative exercise for the body and mind – finding stillness in movement.

The Chinese concept of "chi" is that it is a vital source that animates the body. Learning tai chi is a practical avenue for fostering such things as balance, alignment, fine-scale motor control, rhythm of movement, and more. Thus the practice contributes to health and balance in our lives. In parks across the country now we can see more and more people practicing tai chi, and again there are many free videos available on YouTube.

Aquatic therapy

Aquatic therapy is a specialized form of physical exercise performed in the water. The buoyancy provided by the water is a great benefit, as it assists in supporting the person's weight while submerged and uses the physical properties of water to assist in healing and exercise performance. Buoyancy is the upward thrust acting in the opposite direction than the force of gravity. This therapy reduces the stress placed on the joints, thus making the exercises easier, safer, and less painful to perform, as the buoyancy of the water eliminates up to 90 percent of a person's body weight. The water flow can provide challenges to balance, thus making the practice of balance fun yet safe.

There are physical therapists who now incorporate aquatic work in their therapy. Water therapy has been proven to provide a positive emotional and relaxation state by being in and around water. It is important always to discuss with one's physician before beginning an aquatic therapy program, as for any new form of exercise. What is good for one person is not necessarily recommended for the next. We are individual bodies, each with our own limitations and advantages.

Pilates

Pilates is a series of controlled exercises first implemented by a man named Joseph Pilates. He was hired by the Germans after World War II to help rehabilitate soldiers who had come back from the battlefield. He desired more and left Germany, taking a boat to America, where he founded in New York a system known as controlology. The Pilates method of body conditioning can improve alignment and flexibility, which will encourage proper posture. It is much more than just exercises, however. When it is performed properly, the mind is engaged through deep breathing, which is used to concentrate and to perform the movements. Pilates uses diaphragmatic breathing, which is deep belly breathing where the whole breath is brought into the body, allowing the belly to expand with the inhalation and deflate with the exhalation. This type of abdominal breathing has been said to be the "best practice" of breathing for life in general and is how babies breathe.

The various terms in use today – Pilates mat, Pilates reformer, Pilates chair, PiYo workouts, and others – can make it tough to decide whether it is likely to be suitable for a particular individual. Also, with the deregulation of use of the name Pilates by a court order in the 1990s, there are both knowledgeable and sadly some poor instructors. So as always, be sure to check out the instructor credentials and preview a class before embarking on this journey. The US Pilates Association provides a search engine on its website at www.unitedstatespilatesassociation.com to help locate certified instructors by state. I strongly urge anyone who is interested in learning Pilates mat exercises to find a skilled teacher and take private classes before any group classes, to be sure you learn how the specific movements of the exercises should be done. Your movements will be sharper and your mind will understand more.

Pilates strengthens the main postural muscles, the transverse abdominis. The action of this muscle compresses the abdomen to support the abdominal viscera against the pull of gravity. When these muscles are weak, the lumbar spine can be easily injured. We create a fine-tuned responsiveness to destabilizing forces that enhance balance. Obviously, these are the core muscles much needed in the practice of dentistry for balance and to maintain a neutral position. The Pilates reformer is a machine used to improve flexibility, alignment, and core strength.

Two simple but effective Pilates exercises can help those with and without back problems when performed correctly and consistently: the "single leg stretch" and "rolling back," more commonly called "rolling like a ball." The latter relaxes the spine while scooping of the abdominals strengthens the core. Breathing is what helps keep the momentum going in this fun movement.

TRX

TRX®, which stands for total body resistance exercise, is a revolutionary workout for the total body that uses one's body weight and gravity as resistance to build strength, balance, flexibility, and core and joint stability. A TRX suspension trainer provides wonderful strength training anywhere and anytime, regardless of the individual's fitness level. This total body resistance exercise was invented by a former US Navy Seal. It is a wonderful apparatus to challenge the core, because it uses just two resources, gravity and one's body weight. This system literally let's one hang tough!

Ballet

Ballet is a classical dance form characterized by grace and precision of movement and by elaborate formal gestures, steps, and poses. It has unique traditions and techniques. I mention this classical form here, because the exercises done at the barre are strengthening and promote proper posture and balance when done correctly. I have seen a number of ballet dancers come into the dental school and of course they do not seem to have any problems with correct body positioning, as they know and listen to their body.

Alexander technique

For over 100 years many people have benefited from the Alexander technique, a mind/body process for changing ineffective habits. One learns to release tension, unlock knees, and release breath. Our bad habits place stress on the healthy use and functioning of our whole mind/body system. Using the Alexander technique, range of motion can be greater, tension can be less, and breathing and speaking can be full, natural, and pleasant. A study published in the *British Medical Journal* in 2008 proved the effectiveness of the Alexander technique for pain relief. Rediscover freedom of mind and body with this practice.

Massage therapy and physical therapy

Massage therapists and physical therapists focus individualized programs on therapeutic exercise, which includes strengthening, stretching, patient education, and functional training. Expert chiropractors are also available and should be used to help ease and eliminate problems. Some allied health departments are creating outpatient physical therapy faculties that dental professionals should consider and use as needed on a regular basis.

I see massage therapy as a necessity and not a luxury, as it improves circulation and reduces the internal knots, the "rocks" we get from the daily pressure of work and general living. The trapezius muscles can become elevated over time, causing headaches and shoulder and neck pain. This distress causes the head to "turtle," which is actually the body's protective response to the practitioner's lifting the shoulders and constantly overworking the levator scapular (Figure 7.2). The levator scapulae is one of the muscles of the "motor cylinder" of the neck, which stabilizes muscles deep to the outer sleeves of the trapezius, and its primary function is to elevate the scapulae. We all need an understanding of the stresses the levator itself is working under, which should bring our awareness to the importance of these muscles. The dental operator needs regular muscular manipulation through a scheduled massage at least monthly, if not more frequently, which can help to release the shoulders and to relieve pain (Figures 7.3 and 7.4).

Looking down repetitively can cause strain and overstretching in the occipital region. This can result in chronic headaches and restricted blood flow. The

Figure 7.2 Incorrect working position for the practitioner. Working with raised shoulders causes distress to the spine as the head "turtles" and also causes unnecessary pressure to the wrists, neck, and forearms.

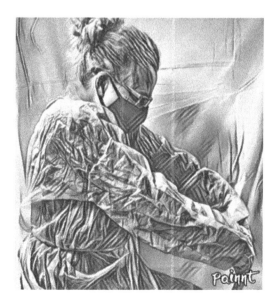

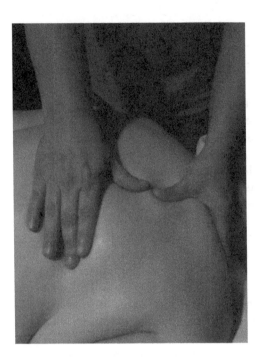

Figure 7.3 Rhomboid along with Trapezius.

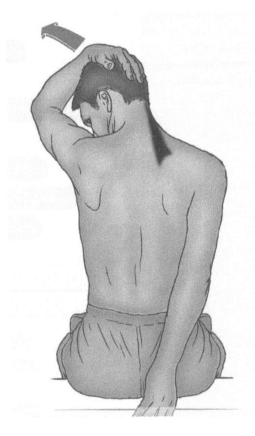

Figure 7.4 The right-side levator scapulae is stretched by flexing, left laterally flexing, and left rotating the neck at the spinal joints, while the right-side should girdle is stabilized downward. *Source:* © Dr. Joe Muscolino (www. learnmuscles.com).

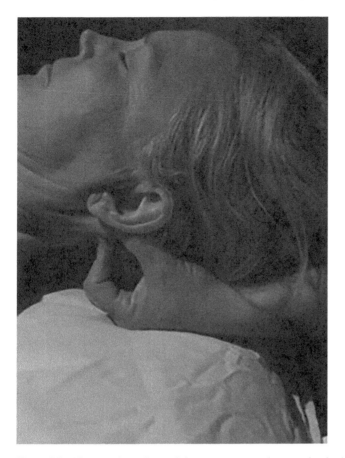

Figure 7.5 Massage therapist applying pressure to reduce tension in the occipital muscles.

massage therapist uses applied pressure in this region that helps relieve tension and improve blood flow to the area (Figure 7.5).

The repetitive flexion of the neck in dentistry can cause shortening of the sternocleidomastoideus (SCM) muscles and overstretching of the posterior cervical muscles, which both contribute to neck misalignment and many other problems. As mentioned previously, the flexion of the neck should be 20 degrees or less. Massage therapy can help here too (Figure 7.6).

Pectoral muscles often become shortened as a result of repetitive shoulder flexion. Using massage to loosen these muscles can help to avoid pain and overstretched muscles in the upper back (Figure 7.7).

About half of all dental professionals unfortunately get low back pain at some point in their career. Lower back pain is often the result of frequent bending over causing the back muscles to remain in an overstretched condition and not

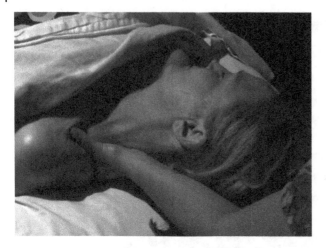

Figure 7.6 Massaging sternocleidomastoid (SCM) clavicle and upper trapezius..

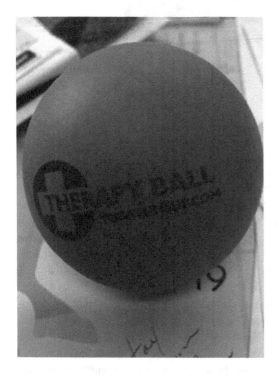

Figure 7.7 Self-massage therapy ball.

Figure 7.8 Easing back pain by massaging the lower back.

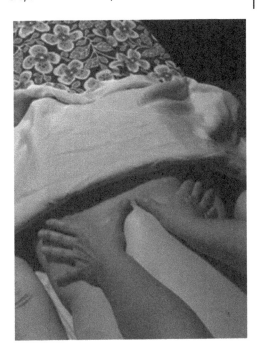

Figure 7.9 Maintaining a neutral wrist position. OK – wrist aligned with long axis of forearm. AVOID – flexion (i.e. bending the wrist and hand down toward the palm).

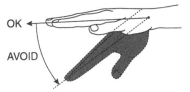

maintaining the normal low back curve. Massage helps to relieve tension and increase blood flow to the area, which in turn helps to bring repair agents or scar tissue to the muscles (Figure 7.8).

Repetitive flexion of the dental practitioner's wrist can cause excessive inflammation to the flexor reticulum, which leads to carpal tunnel syndrome (Figures 7.9 and 7.10).

The Craniosacral System

The craniosacral system has recently been recognized as a functioning physiological system. It involves the meningeal membranes, the osseous structures to which the meningeal membranes attach, the nonosseous connective tissue structures that are intimately related to the meningeal membranes, the cerebrospinal fluid, and all structures related to production, resorption, and containment of the cerebrospinal fluid.

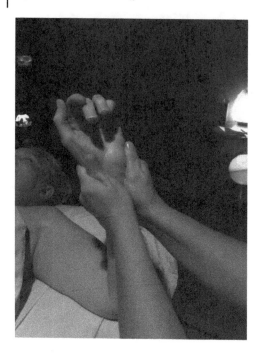

Figure 7.10 Therapy for the flexor reticulum.

This system is influenced by the nervous system, the musculoskeletal system, the vascular and lymphatic systems, and the endocrine and respiratory systems. Abnormalities in the structure or function of any of these systems may influence the craniosacral system. This massage therapy uses the operator's palpatory skills with a very light touch of the hands to follow the craniosacral motion and correct the eventual restrictions, allowing the system to "auto-correct." Light touch is used to examine the membranes and movement of the fluids in and around the central nervous system. This relieves tension in the central nervous system and promotes a feeling of well-being by eliminating pain and boosting immunity. This delicate technique works deeply on the nervous system, giving the body both psychological and emotional harmony, and can bring benefits in many ways to the individual.

Taking a break

A day in the life of a dental practitioner is filled with constant energy expended on preparing to give excellent patient care. Practitioners must keep in mind the need to incorporate practice breaks in their day. Stand up and stretch each side of the body. Reach to the sky. Do chairside stretching. Roll the neck carefully from one shoulder to the other. Shake out the body and just let go! Do thigh- or ankle-strengthening exercises (Figures 7.11 and 7.12). Go to a private place and do a cat/cow stretch or

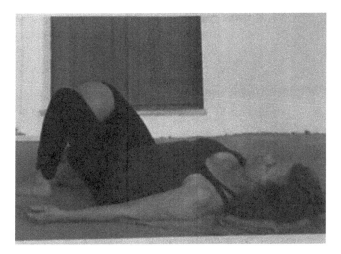

Figure 7.11   Thigh-strengthening exercise.

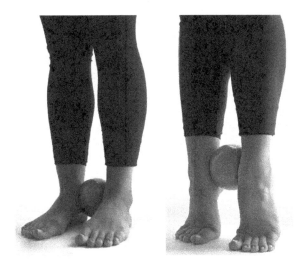

Figure 7.12   Using a yoga therapy ball.

the "child's pose" from yoga to relax the lower back, or do some deep breathing. An easy example of using the breath to calm the emotions and thus the physical body is to inhale slowly for 8 counts using the diaphragm to expand the rib cage, then to hold the breath for 7 or 8 counts, and then to exhale slowly for 8 counts. This breathing can be calming as well as energizing. Meditate by looking out of the window at the blue sky for a few minutes and relax, enjoy, and empty the mind. Taking a break can help dental practitioners to better handle work-related stress. Also remember to eat right, keep a good attitude, and smile.

8

Red Flags

An ounce of prevention is worth a pound of cure

The red flag is a warning of moving into an unhealthy area or level. For the dental practitioner, encountering a red flag should be a significant moment to stop and figure out the problem to turn life around and move toward health and liberation.

Tingling, numbness, shoulder freeze, low back pain, stiff neck, swollen knees, aching forearms, and/or general fatigue and discomfort are all red flags that should alert the dental practitioner that something is wrong. Stop here and begin to figure out what movements are provoking the pain. What is the nature of the pain? Is the pain constant and unremitting? Is morning stiffness a daily occurrence? This is the time to have an appropriate consultation with a good doctor or physical therapist. Find the cause to prevent the damage.

One owes it to oneself to remember to thy own self be true. A wonderful dental career can be had for practitioners who wisely use their insight with patience and discipline to find and use the proper positioning of the body for every moment of practice.

Ergonomics in the Dental Office, First Edition. Susan S. Parker.
© 2022 John Wiley & Sons, Inc. Published 2022 by John Wiley & Sons, Inc.

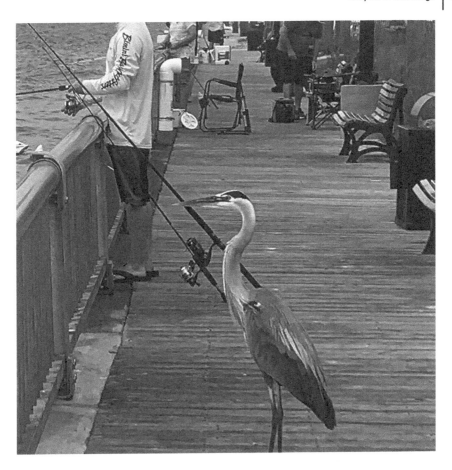

THE DIFFERENCE BETWEEN WHO YOU ARE AND WHO YOU WANT TO BE... IS WHAT YOU DO.

Bibliography

Academy of General Dentistry, www.agd.org.

Ahearn, D.J. (2005) The eight keys to selecting great seating for long-term health. *Dentistry Today*, September 1. Retrieved August 23, 2021 from http://www.dentistrytoday.com/ergonomics/1115--sp-1633235012.

American Dental Association, www.ada.org.

Bhattachanye, A., & McGlothlin, J. (2012) *Occupational Ergonomics: Theory and Application*. Boca Raton, FL: CRC Press.

Biel, A. (2001) *Trail Guide to the Body*, 2nd edn. Boulder, CO: Books of Discovery.

Bridger, R. (2004) *An Introduction to Ergonomics*, 2nd edn. Boca Raton, FL: CRC Press.

Costco Connection. January 2021. Retrieved September 15, 2021 from https://www.costcoconnection.com/connection/202101/.

Dental Lifeline Network, www.dentallifeline.org.

Dimensions of Dental Hygiene, www.dimensionsofdentalhygiene.com.

Elsenpeter, R. (2017) How better dental office design can prolong your career. *Dental Products Report*, May 12. Retrieved August 23, 2021 from http://www.dentalproductsreport.com/dental/article/how-better-dental-office-design-can-prolong-your-career.

Finkbeiner, B.L. (2014) The biggest ergonomic mistakes dental professionals make. *Dental Products Report*, August 27. www. Retrieved September 28, 2017 from https://www.dentalproductsreport.com/view/biggest-ergonomic-mistakes-dental-professionals-make.

Finkbeiner, B.L., & Muscari, M. (2006) Let ergonomics and true four-handed dentistry help you. *Dentistry IQ*, June 1. Retrieved August 23, 2021 from http://www.dentistryiq.com/articles/dem/print/volume-11/issue-3/equipment/let-ergonomics-and-true-four-handed-dentistry-help-you.

García-Vidal, J.A., López-Nicolás, M., Sánchez-Sobrado, A.C. et al. (2019) The combination of different ergonomic supports during dental procedures reduces muscle activity of the neck and shoulder. *Journal of Clinical Medicine*, 8(8): 1230.

Gupta, A., Ankola, A.V., & Hebbal, M. (2015) Dental ergonomics to combat musculoskeletal disorders. *International Journal of Occupational Safety and Ergonomics*, 36(5): 561–571.

Gupta, A., Bhat, M., Mohammed, T., Bansal, N., & Gupta, G. (2014) Ergonomics in dentistry. *International Journal of Clinical Pediatric Dentistry*, 7(1): 730–733.

Gupta, S. (2011) Ergonomic applications to dental practice. *Indian Journal of Dental Research*, 22(6): 816–822.

Hayes, M.J., Smith, D.R., & Cockrell, D. (2009) A systemic review of musculoskeletal disorders among dental professionals. *International Dental Journal*, 7(3): 159–165.

Holt, E., & Hoebeka, R. (2012) How illumination can improve your musculoskeletal health. *Dimensions of Dental Hygiene*, Sept.

Holstein, W.K., & Chapanis, A. (2018). Human-factors engineering. *Encyclopedia Britannica*. Retrieved August 23, 2021 from https://www.britannica.com/topic/human-factors-engineering.

Jacobs, K. (2008) *Ergonomics for Therapists*, 3rd edn. Philadelphia, PA: Mosby Elsevier.

Jones, A.C. (2005) Functional training for dentistry: An exercise for dental health care personnel. *CDA Journal*, 33(2): 137–145.

Khan, M.J., & Chew, K.Y. (2013) Effect of working characteristics and taught ergonomics on the prevalence of musculoskeletal disorders amongst dental students. *BMC Musculoskeletal Disorders*, 14: 118.

Ligh, R.Q. (2002) Preventing cumulative trauma injury – carpal tunnel syndrome. *CDA Journal*, 30: 671.

Matsuda, S. (2012) The dynamics of pressure. *Dimensions of Dental Hygiene*, Sept.

Merriam-Webster. (n.d.). Ergonomics. *Merriam-Webster.com Dictionary*. Retrieved August 23, 2021 from https://www.merriam-webster.com/dictionary/ergonomics.

Murphy, D. (ed.) (1998) *Ergonomics and the Dental Care Worker*. Washington, DC: American Public Health Association.

Muscolino, J. (n.d.) Anatomy Encyclopedia. *Learn Muscles*. Retrieved August 23, 2021 from https://learnmuscles.com/glossary.

Nunn, P. Posture for dental hygiene practice. In D. Murphy (ed.), *Ergonomics and the Dental Care Worker*. Washington, DC: American Public Health Association.

Occupational Health and Safety Administration, www.osha.gov.

OH&S (2020) The relationship between MSDs and the workplace. *Occupational Health and Safety*, Feb 13. Retrieved September 15, 2021 from https://ohsonline.com/articles/2020/02/13/the-relationship-between-msds-and-the-workplace.aspx.

Parker, S. (2010a) The core of ergonomic practice. *Dimensions of Dental Hygiene*, Jan: 36–37.

Parker, S. (2010b) The Pilates approach to back pain. *Dimensions of Dental Hygiene*, April: 52–53.

Phebus, J.G. (2015) Why ergonomics should be emphasized in dental school curricula. *Compendium of Continuing Education in Dentistry*, 36(5).

Pollack, S. (2002) *All the Right Moves*. Tulsa, OK: PennWell Books.

Procter & Gamble, www.dentalcare.com.

Shrivardhan, K., Kakarla, V.V.P., Kumar, G.C., Shravani, D., & Chaya, C. (2014) Insights into ergonomics among dental professionals of a dental institute and private practitioners in Hubli-Dharwad Twin Cities, India. *Safety and Health at Work*, 5(4): 181–185.

Thornton, L.J., Barr, A., Stuart-Buttle, C. et al. (2008) Perceived musculoskeletal symptoms among dental students in the clinic environment. *Journal of Ergonomics*, 51(4): 573–586.

United Cerebral Palsy, www.ucp.org.

United States Ergonomics, www.us-ergo.com

US Department of Health and Human Services, www.hhs.gov.

Valachi, B. (2009) Ergonomic guidelines for selecting patient chairs and delivery systems. *Dentistry Today*, July 1. Retrieved August 23, 2021 from http://www.dentistrytoday.com/ergonomics/1112-Sp-52800858.

Valachi, B., & Valachi, K. (2003) Preventing musculoskeletal disorders in clinical dentistry. *Journal of the American Dental Association*, 134(12): 1604–1612.

Wann, O., & Canull, B. (2003) Ergonomics and dental hygienists. *Contemporary Oral Hygiene*, 3(5): 15–22.

Index

Ergonomics in the Dental Office, First Edition. Susan S. Parker.
© 2022 John Wiley & Sons, Inc. Published 2022 by John Wiley & Sons, Inc.